the little book of

AROMATHERAPY

Published by OH!
20 Mortimer Street
London W1T 3JW

Disclaimer:
This book and the information contained herein are for general
educational and entertainment use only. The contents are not claimed to
be exhaustive, and the book is sold on the understanding that neither the
publishers nor the author are thereby engaged in rendering any kind of
professional services. Users are encouraged to confirm the information
contained herein with other sources and review the information
carefully with their appropriate, qualified service providers. Neither the
publishers nor the author shall have any responsibility to any person
or entity regarding any loss or damage whatsoever, direct or indirect,
consequential, special or exemplary, caused or alleged to be caused, by
the use or misuse of information contained in this book.

ISBN 978-1-91161-085-4

Editorial consultant: Sasha Fenton
Editorial: Angela Mogridge, Victoria Godden
Project manager: Russell Porter
Design: Ben Ruocco
Production: Rachel Burgess

A CIP catalogue record for this book is available from the British Library

Printed in China

10 9 8 7 6 5 4 3

the little book of
AROMATHERAPY

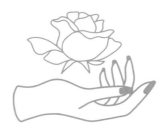

angela mogridge

CONTENTS

"Aromatherapy is a caring,
first-hand therapy that seeks
to induce relaxation,
to increase energy, to reduce
the effects of stress and to
restore lost balance to mind,
body and soul."

ROBERT TISSERAND

WHAT IS AROMATHERAPY?

Aromatherapy is a form of alternative medicine that uses the oils from plants to enhance physical and psychological well-being.

Essential oils, as they are known, are taken from flowers, barks, stems, leaves and roots. Each of the oils has its own unique healing properties and fragrance, and several oils can be combined for maximum effect.

Aromatherapy is often referred to as a form of *holistic therapy* or *medicine* because it is used to heal the whole person – the body, spirit and emotions.

INTRODUCTION

6

IMPORTANT NOTE

All complementary therapies can be useful, but anyone who has a health problem must consult a medical doctor and take the medicines and treatments that are prescribed. Some complementary therapies, such as aromatherapy, will cause problems to those who are also taking conventional medication.

Always read the instructions that come with any medicine, whether it has been prescribed by a doctor or bought over the counter.

CHAPTER

1

ABOUT
AROMA

Smell is the most powerful of our senses. As it is the only sense connected to the brain's limbic system, it can trigger powerful memories and emotional responses.

This fact is not lost on marketing companies – a petrol station experiment saw a 300% increase in drink sales when the smell of coffee was pumped through the air conditioning.

"Smell is a potent wizard that transports us across thousands of miles and all the years we have lived."

HELEN KELLER

DID YOU KNOW?

- It takes petals from thirty roses to produce one drop of rose essential oil

- Several kilos of lavender flowers are needed to produce a bottle of lavender essential oil

- The Bible references essential oils over 150 times as a means of healing

- Essential oils are safer to use to clean your house than chemicals, which can cause exposure to toxins

"Humanity will be saved through the flower."

HUVENOL, MAYAN ELDER

NOTES from HISTORY

In 3500 BC, Egyptian priestesses were burning frankincense to clear the mind, while the Romans used various essential oils for massage. In 17th-century England, wealthy people who had to walk through smelly neighbourhoods would hold pomanders of oranges and cloves to their noses. Some people used herbs in face masks to ward off the plague, sweating sickness and other viruses. It was a French chemist – René-Maurice Gattefossé – who coined the term aromatherapy in 1937 to describe our modern-day usage of the oils.

"Imagine a survivor of a failed civilisation with only a tattered book on aromatherapy for guidance in arresting a cholera epidemic. Yet such a book would more likely be found amongst the debris than a comprehensive medical text."

JAMES LOVELOCK

HOW
to use
ESSENTIAL OILS

Perhaps the most relaxing and effective way of using aromatherapy oils is through massage. Two or three oils, blended with a carrier oil such as almond, are combined with massage techniques so that they can be absorbed through the skin into the bloodstream. You can learn self-massage techniques, or you can visit a qualified therapist.

The easiest way to experience the benefits of aromatherapy is to add a few drops of essential oil to your bathwater. Light a candle, lie back and luxuriate while relaxing to the smells of jasmine or rose or ylang-ylang. Why not rub a little cedarwood or clary sage into your scalp just before you climb into the bath for the ultimate in self-care?

Need help clearing the sinuses? Eucalyptus, thyme, lemon and tea tree are all good oils to help ease colds, sniffles and sneezes. They are known for their antibacterial properties, and work well. Simply add five drops of your chosen essential oil to a bowl of boiling water, put a towel over your head like a tent and breathe in.

Have a headache that won't go away?
How about sore muscles from that trip to
the gym? Does your tummy hurt? Add a few
drops of oil to a bowl of warm water, soak
a flannel in the water, wring it out and use it
as a compress on the area that hurts. Give
peppermint, lavender or chamomile a try.

Aromatherapy doesn't just work when applied
to the body. You can use essential oils to
fragrance a room to create a certain mood or
ambience. Oils are often added to candles, and
as the wax melts, they release their smell. You
can also use an oil burner or reed diffuser to
evaporate and distribute the aroma.

"Aromatherapy is
extremely useful.
If you want to go to
sleep at night, and you
have an aroma that
calms your mind, it will
help you sleep."

DEEPAK CHOPRA

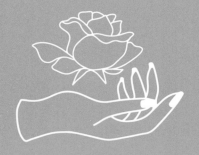

CHAPTER

2

a list of
ESSENTIAL
OILS

As you have probably guessed, there is an almost infinite number of essential oils, each one with an equally endless list of benefits.

By using one on its own or two or three blended together, you can create your own aromatherapy remedy for whatever is ailing you at the time – a unique blend for your individual, unique needs.

*"They are much
to be pitied who have
not been given
a taste for nature
early in life."*

JANE AUSTEN

BASIL

Basil is known as the oil of renewal. It is distilled from the cooking herb, and it has a sweet, spicy, almost liquorice aroma. It improves mental clarity, clears the mind and is useful for soothing exam or interview nerves.

It blends well with geranium, bergamot and any citrus oils. It has even been claimed that basil can help people who are overcoming addiction. Only use this oil in small amounts.

Basil can also be useful for:

	Headaches
	Sinus congestion
	Fainting
	Fatigued or sore muscles
	Anxiety and fear
	Mental clarity and memory
	Concentration
	Exhaustion
	Lack of direction
	Nervousness

BERGAMOT

Bergamot is often referred to as the oil of self-acceptance. Extracted from the peel of a small orange-like fruit, bergamot has a sweet, citrus aroma. This light and uplifting fragrance blends well with many other oils and is often used in massage due to its calming and soothing properties. It is especially helpful to those who struggle with self-love and self-worth, and it can even help that "Monday morning feeling".

Note: Bergamot oil should not be used within three hours of going out in the sun or when using a sunbed.

Bergamot can also be useful for:

	Supporting the digestive system
	Depression
	PMT
	Anxiety
	Shyness
	Stress
	Skin rejuvenation
	Lack of confidence
	Regret
	Despondency
	Travel sickness
	Worry

BENZOIN

Benzoin is a thick resin-oil that is golden in colour with a vanilla-like aroma. Benzoin is warming, soothing and penetrating.

Its properties are antidepressant, antiseptic, anti-inflammatory and anti-rheumatic. It blends well with orange, coriander, frankincense, bergamot, juniper, lavender, myrrh, rose, lemon and sandalwood oils.

Benzoin can also be useful for:

	Improving circulation
	Preventing sepsis
	Improving digestion
	Blisters
	Depression
	Anxiety
	Removing bad odours
	Protecting open wounds from infection
	Arthritis
	Coughs
	Chapped, cracked or dry skin
	Loneliness
	Tension and nervousness
	Sadness

BLACK PEPPER

Associated with clarity and honesty, black pepper enables people to share their true feelings and emotions. Black pepper is one of the oldest known spices, and it is a very stimulating essential oil. It is a rich source of antioxidants which aids digestion and blood circulation. With a very sharp and spicy aroma, it blends well with basil, bergamot, frankincense, geranium and rosemary. It dilates blood vessels, too, which is good for easing aches and pains.

Black pepper can also be useful for:

	Constipation
	Muscle aches
	Sickness
	Digestive problems
	Flu
	Fevers
	Stomach pains
	Anxiety

CAJUPUT

Cajuput has a sweet, penetrating aroma and is often found in cosmetics and perfume. It has strong antiseptic properties and is widely described as an anti-spasmodic, analgesic and decongestant oil.

Cajuput can also be useful for:

	Colds
	Bronchitis
	Sinusitis
	Dysentery
	Arthritis and rheumatism

	Acne
	Insect bites
	Headache, earache, toothache
	Cynicism
	Improving memory
	Laryngitis
	Asthma
	Colic
	Vomiting
	Muscular aches and pains
	Psoriasis
	Gout
	Compulsiveness
	Disorientation
	Procrastination

CAMPHOR

Camphor is a powerful and volatile oil that has a sharp, pungent and piercing odour. It is often used in pharmaceutical medicines for conditions such as cardiac failure. For more everyday usage, camphor oil is suitable for anyone suffering from colds or flu. Camphor is warming and thus is perfect for use during winter. It can be used as a steam inhalant with a few drops dissolved in hot water to help soothe a cold or sinus infection. It is also useful as an antiseptic for insect bites, or even as an insect repellent if used in a candle or diffuser.

Note: Camphor must be used in tiny dosages as it can be toxic.

"Bread feeds
the body, indeed,
but flowers
feed also the soul."

THE KORAN

CARDAMOM

Cardamom has an intense, spicy, warming aroma that is sometimes likened to mint. A popular cooking spice, especially in Indian food, it is also used in powder form to regulate high blood pressure. In terms of aromatherapy, cardamom is used for digestive problems and even food poisoning due to its antibacterial properties. Cardamom is seen as an invigorating and expanding essential oil. It is often used psychologically for outbursts of anger, rage or frustration, and it can help a person see a situation more clearly.

Note: Cardamom should not be used on babies or children.

Cardamom can also be useful for:

	Colic (in adults)
	Fungal infections
	Anxiety
	Mood disorders
	Stomach upsets
	Indigestion
	Asthma
	Confusion
	Selfishness
	Respiratory health

CEDARWOOD

Cedarwood essential oil is said to have a calming, grounding effect on the nervous system. On a spiritual level, it brings people together. It has a pleasant, woody, smoky aroma that blends well with bergamot, frankincense, jasmine, lavender, neroli and rose. Users often find that cedarwood instils a sense of peace, and it is favoured by those who meditate. Cedarwood stimulates the lymphatic system, which makes it excellent for respiratory conditions such as catarrh, asthma or bronchitis.

Note: Cedarwood should not be used during pregnancy.

Cedarwood can also be useful for:

	Urinary tract conditions
	Burning pains
	Oily skin
	Acne
	Chronic skin conditions
	Vaginal infections and discharges
	Itching
	Dandruff
	Cellulite
	Scattered thoughts

CHAMOMILE

Roman chamomile oil is distilled from the flowers of the chamomile plant and has a fruity, apple-like aroma. It is a good one for the first-aid box as it is anti-inflammatory, soothing and very versatile.

It blends particularly well with bergamot, clary sage, geranium, jasmine, lavender, sandalwood and ylang-ylang. Spiritually, chamomile is said to bring peace, love and acceptance and to encourage a sense of purposefulness. It is also useful when dealing with grief and shock.

Physically, chamomile is helpful for:

	Muscular pain
	Use as a sedative
	Chilblains
	Dermatitis
	Nettle rash
	Anxiety and tension
	Bedwetting
	Colic
	Hot flushes
	Rheumatoid arthritis

CINNAMON

Cinnamon has an earthy, spicy aroma. In oil form, it smells more peppery and muskier than ground cinnamon.

Cinnamon oil revives and stimulates the body and the senses. Traditionally cinnamon has been used as a remedy for digestive problems. It blends well with orange and clove oils but can irritate the skin, so should be used with caution. Cinnamon oil can also be useful for:

	Colds and flu
	Shivering cold
	Aches and pains

	Lack of creativity
	Feelings of weakness
	Mental exhaustion
	Emotional coldness
	Dental pain
	Wasp stings, snake bites, lice
	Fevers
	Infections
	Diabetes
	Feelings of isolation and loneliness
	Fear
	Depression
	Menstrual problems
	Strengthening the heart and nervous system
	Lack of concentration

*"Oils of cinnamon
and eucalyptus are as
powerful against some
micro-organisms as
conventional antibiotics,
and are especially effective
against flu."*

ROBERT TISSERAND

"I am big into aromatherapy."

SHARON STONE

CITRONELLA

If you have ever lit a little yellow candle
on a hotel balcony in a bid to ward off
mosquitoes, then you will already be aware
of citronella and its sweet, lemony aroma.

As well as an insect repellent, citronella is
also a popular ingredient in deodorants,
air fresheners, fabric fresheners and even
foot sprays. Citronella blends well with
other members of the citrus family such as
grapefruit, lemon, lime, orange, petitgrain
and mandarin.

"I believe that essential oils may someday prove a vital weapon in the fight against strains of antibiotic-resistant bacteria."

ANDREW WEIL

CLARY SAGE

Clary sage is an excellent all-purpose oil, which is often used in aromatherapy massage. It has a warm, nutty, woody smell which some people compare to the aroma of warm hay. The properties of clary sage are a magic mixture of stimulation, balance and inspiration as well as being sensual and peaceful. It is great when blended with jasmine, geranium, sandalwood, bergamot and frankincense.

Note: You should avoid using clary sage when taking medicines containing iron or when drinking alcohol.

Clary sage can also be useful for:

	Exhaustion and insomnia
	Claustrophobia

	Relaxation
	Stress
	Hostility
	Negative thoughts and depression
	Hair loss
	Impotence
	Wounds
	Addiction
	PMT
	Compulsiveness
	Over-work
	Listlessness
	Melancholy
	Mid-life crises
	Digestive and stomach problems

CLOVE

Clove oil is a powerful antiseptic that is traditionally associated with the relief of toothache. It is anti-inflammatory and pain-relieving, making it an excellent addition to the first-aid kit. It does have a strong fragrance which is not to everyone's taste, but its benefits to the liver, skin and mouth make up for this.

Note: Clove essential oil is potent and concentrated, so it is best administered by a professional aromatherapist.

Clove can also be useful for:

	Toothache
	Candida and thrush
	Protecting against bacteria and viruses
	Travel sickness
	Flatulence
	Boosting the immune system
	Slowing down skin ageing
	Indigestion
	Bloating
	Stomach ulcers

CORIANDER

With a sweet yet spicy aroma, coriander is stimulating and refreshing. It is a well-known cooking spice, and its oil is distilled from its seeds. Coriander is a powerful agent which blends well with bergamot, cinnamon, grapefruit, ginger, neroli, orange, lime and lemon.

Due to its antibacterial qualities, coriander is sometimes used in deodorants and mouthwashes. Coriander essential oil can be used as a relaxant, a stimulant, and to support the digestive and hormonal systems.

Coriander can also be useful for:

	Lack of appetite
	Digestive problems
	Lack of energy
	A busy mind
	Oily skin
	Stomach pain and upset
	Painful joints and muscles
	Lack of motivation
	Self-acceptance

CYPRESS

Cypress essential oil is distilled from the leaves and cones of the tree. It is commonly used to fight infection, remove toxins from the body, aid the digestive system and relax the nerves.

It makes a particularly effective footbath due to its astringent properties.

Cypress can also be useful for:

	Healing wounds and infections
	Inflammation and water retention
	Cleansing the liver
	Lowering cholesterol levels
	Anxiety
	Reducing frequent urination
	Muscle cramps and restless leg syndrome
	Improving circulation
	Preventing acne
	Respiratory conditions and asthma
	Insomnia
	Bronchitis coughs

EUCALYPTUS

Eucalyptus warms the body in winter and cools it in the summer. It is stimulating and balancing and has powerful antiseptic properties. Originally from Australia, Aboriginal people view the plant and oil as a cure for a myriad of conditions. The koala bear feeds only on eucalyptus leaves, and many Australians smoke the leaves to relieve asthma.

Eucalyptus oil is often added to sauna coals or steam room sprinklers in spas. The aroma of eucalyptus can overwhelm other essential oils, so it is mainly used on its own rather than in a blend.

Particularly helpful for the respiratory
system and a potent antifungal,
antiseptic and antiviral, eucalyptus oil
can also be useful for:

	Asthma and bronchitis
	Sinusitis
	Fevers
	Colds, catarrh, flu and congestion
	Headaches
	Diabetes

"The Earth laughs in flowers."

RALPH WALDO EMERSON

*"Their fruit
will be for food,
and their leaves
for healing."*

EZEKIEL 47:12

FENNEL

A traditional cooking herb, fennel has a strong liquorice flavour and aroma. It was favoured by the Romans and said to promote strength, courage and longevity. Fennel essential oil blends well with basil, geranium, lavender, lemon, rosemary and sandalwood. It should be used with caution during pregnancy and avoided entirely if you have a history of seizures. Fennel is well-known for its digestion-calming and hormone-balancing properties and can also be useful for:

	Stomachaches
	Bloating and wind

	Excessive appetite
	Nausea
	Minor skin irritations
	Regulating menstrual cycles
	Easing menstual pain
	Lack of motivation
	Healing wounds
	Low self-esteem and self-doubt
	Indigestion
	Colic
	Cellulite
	Stubbornness
	Preventing stomach spasms
	Increasing stamina
	Constipation

FRANKINCENSE

Frankincense is a rejuvenating oil with a warm, spicy scent that is often used in meditation. Its incense-like intoxicating aroma has long made it the go-to essential oil for anyone wanting to feel nurtured. With a long history of being used in religious ceremonies and rituals, frankincense is now used in medicine and in expensive perfumes and potions.

With strong anti-inflammatory properties, it stimulates the nervous system. In addition, it can be used for its calming effects during childbirth.

Frankincense can also be useful for:

	Nosebleeds
	Acne scarring
	Urinary tract infections
	Wounds, ulcers and skin inflammation
	Claustrophobia
	Irritability
	Haemorrhoids
	Colds
	Pain management
	Bereavement
	Fear and apprehension
	Nerves

GERANIUM

With a fresh but strong and heavy rose-like scent, geranium is widely used in the production of expensive perfumes and cosmetics.

Geranium is known as a balancing oil, as it is capable of both uplifting and sedating a user. It helps relieve fear and depression while also soothing anxiety and tension. Balancing, detoxifying, regulating and decongesting – there isn't much this wonder oil can't do!

Geranium can also be useful for:

	Hormone balancing
	PMT
	Boosting the immune system
	Calming the mind
	Mood swings
	Stomach upsets
	Stabilizing blood pressure
	Throat and mouth infections
	Menopause
	Dermatitis
	Stress
	Rigidity
	Treating wounds
	Urinary, liver or circulatory disorders

GINGER

Produced from the root of the ginger plant, this oil is a renowned aphrodisiac. Ginger also has a range of pharmaceutical and medical uses in addition to the distinct culinary and beverage uses. It is a potent oil that should only be used in small amounts.

Ginger blends well with other oils including cardamom, cinnamon, clove, eucalyptus and frankincense. Citrus oils, such as lemon, lime and orange, also work well with ginger. Ginger is warming, healing and strengthening, and it can settle the digestive system.

Ginger can also be useful for:

	Headaches
	Muscle pains
	Cramps
	Male impotence
	Arthritis
	Fatigue
	Colds and flu

GRAPEFRUIT

With a tangy, fresh, fruity aroma, grapefruit essential oil is uplifting and refreshing. Physically, grapefruit can help suppress the appetite and increase the metabolism, so it is therefore useful for digestive problems.

Grapefruit essential oil helps to detoxify the system while calming the mind and is thus a valuable aid to any stress-related ailments such as:

	Bitterness
	Lack of clarity
	Despondency
	Negativity
	Depression
	General stress
	Envy or jealousy
	Procrastination
	Frustration

"*Healing begins
with an aromatic
bath and
daily massage.*"

HIPPOCRATES

"The physician heals; nature makes well."

ARISTOTLE

HYSSOP

Hyssop has a purifying scent that can be described as minty and flowery. It is a powerful essence that is best used by a qualified aromatherapist.

It is an anti-inflammatory, antioxidant essential oil which has uplifting properties.

Hyssop can also be useful for:

	Colds, coughs and sore throats
	Hypertension
	Inflammation
	Skin irritation
	Eczema and psoriasis
	Asthma and respiratory problems
	Hypotension
	Infections
	Minor bites and small cuts
	Grief

JASMINE

Known as the king of the essential oils, jasmine is one of the most expensive aromatherapy oils on the market. Its fragrance is exotic, flowery, almost honey-like, making it a favourite massage oil.

This oil revitalizes and uplifts, replacing negativity with positivity and sadness with joy. It is capable of changing moods swiftly and dramatically. Jasmine is said to increase intuitive wisdom, open up a subject emotionally and even develop psychic ability. This will make the individual more receptive to love, trust and happiness.

Jasmine can also be useful for:

	Apathy
	Sadness and depression
	Stress and tension
	Lack of confidence
	Nervous exhaustion
	Shyness
	Apprehension about the future
	Detachment
	Negativity
	Post-natal depression
	Paranoia
	Fear
	Emotional expression

JUNIPER

Distilled from the berries, juniper essential oil has excellent purifying and cleansing properties. It clears the spirit and rejuvenates the body. With a hot, smoky, balsamic aroma, juniper has been described as smelling like gin or even turpentine. It is often used for cleansing and purifying a room before meditation.

Both stimulating and relaxing at the same time, juniper can uplift you in times of challenge or stress.

Juniper can also be useful for:

	Swelling caused by arthritis
	Hangovers
	Hayfever
	Lethargy
	Worry
	Stiff limbs
	Dermatitis, acne and other skin complaints
	Cramps
	Water retention
	Cystitis
	Fear and anxiety
	Difficulty sleeping
	Bad breath

"If you had to choose an oil, it would have to be lavender essential oil, because it is antibacterial and antiviral. So, it's great to have when people around you are sick; it can also be used to relax."

KAREN ROSE

"*I put a drop of lavender essential oil on my pillow before I go to sleep.*"

MELISSA JOAN HART

LAVENDER

The best known of the essential oils, lavender is the most versatile oil and an essential part of any first-aid kit. Its soothing aroma is instantly recognizable, and it is often used in cosmetic and perfume production. The main ingredient in potpourri, lavender is also used to keep insects at bay and to keep drawers smelling fresh. Lavender oil is calming, soothing and balancing both physically and emotionally.

Lavender can also be useful for:

	Earache
	Insomnia
	Nausea and migraines

	Arthritis
	Fear
	Mood swings
	Worry
	Insect bites
	Acne and eczema
	Chilblains
	Indigestion
	Bruises and nosebleeds
	Exhaustion
	Hysteria and negative thoughts
	Sore and swollen joints
	Hot flushes
	Skin burns
	Restlessness

"You can place a drop of lavender oil on your hands and let your dog pick up the scent. It is best to do this in association with pleasant experiences, such as feeding time and before walks. Do this as often as possible. The positive association will allow it to calm down and remain relaxed."

CESAR MILLAN

"I only use essential oils for perfumes."

JESSICA CAPSHAW

LEMON

Produced from the rind of the fruit, 3,000 lemons are needed to produce a kilo of oil. It is another essential addition to the first-aid kit due to its antibacterial, antiseptic and germicidal properties.

It is a top-rated essential oil in Japan, where it is believed to boost brain power and productivity. Lemon oil can also be used to remove oil or grease spots on clothing and can even function as bleach on fair hair and freckles.

Lemon can also be useful for:

	Verrucas and warts
	Sore throats
	Strengthening the immune system
	Bleeding
	Stomach infections
	Fevers
	Colds and flu
	Anaemia
	Swelling
	Circulatory disorders

LEMONGRASS

With an aroma resembling lemon sherbet, this is a popular essential oil for use in perfumes. The oil is extracted from the leaves and stalks of the lemongrass plant, but it also has significant antibacterial properties. It is often found in soaps and face cleansers, while in aromatherapy it helps relieve depression, anxiety and stress.

Lemongrass can also be used as an effective insect repellent. As well as its antibacterial properties, lemongrass is anti-inflammatory, antifungal and an antioxidant.

Lemongrass can also be useful for:

	Athlete's foot
	Stomach pain
	Dehydration
	High cholesterol
	Stress and anxiety
	Muscle aches and pains
	Gingivitis
	Nausea
	Diarrhoea
	Headaches and migraines
	Boredom and lack of interest

MANDARIN

With a refreshing, cooling and exotic aroma, mandarin essential oil smells just like the fruit from which it is taken.

It is gentle yet strengthening, calming yet uplifting, revitalizing and inspiring.

Mandarin can also be useful for:

	PMT
	Morning sickness
	Digestive problems
	Scaring
	Depression
	Appetite
	Hiccups
	Stretchmarks
	Anxiety
	Insomnia

MARJORAM

With a warm, peppery, penetrating smell, marjoram promotes health and well-being and is known for its warming properties. Marjoram blends well with bergamot, cardamom, clary sage and frankincense. There are different types of marjoram, and it is vital to only use sweet marjoram for aromatherapy purposes.

Marjoram relaxes the brain and calms the nervous system. It has also been used throughout history to cover unpleasant odours – being used as a nosegay in Stuart times.

Note: Marjoram should not be used during pregnancy.

Marjoram can also be useful for:

	Chills
	Mental strain
	Hysteria
	Hyperactivity
	Overwork
	Muscle spasms, aches and strains
	Anxiety and nervous tension
	Hostility
	Irrational thoughts

MELISSA

Melissa essential oil has a fragrant, lemony scent, and it is often referred to as lemon balm. It is commonly used in skin balms due to its soothing properties. Melissa has been called the "elixir of life" because of its ability to lift the mood, drive away sadness and promote joy and an overall feeling of wellness.

Note: Melissa should be avoided if pregnant or if you have sensitive skin.

Melissa can also be useful for:

	Colds
	Vertigo
	Apprehension about the future
	PMT
	Insomnia
	Spasms
	Digestive problems
	High blood pressure
	Nerves
	Shock
	Anxiety and nervous tension
	Inflammation
	Bloating
	Bacterial infections
	Fevers

MYRRH

Myrrh essential oil is distilled from the dried sap of the thorny myrrh tree. Its amber-coloured oil has an earthy smell, and it is one of the oldest essential oils. It has long been used in Chinese traditional medicine, Ayurvedic medicine and aromatherapy. Myrrh has strong religious significance for many people.

During biblical times, myrrh incense was burned at sacred sites to help purify the air. It was always carried by Greek soldiers into battle to treat their wounds. Myrrh blends well with frankincense, lemon and lavender.

Myrrh can also be useful:

	Dry coughs
	Throat infections
	Headaches
	Joint pain
	Mouth infections
	Wounds
	Back pain

NEROLI

Also known as orange blossom, neroli is the first-choice essential oil for stress, shock and depression. Its scent has variously been described as exquisite, cooling, refreshing, exhilarating, enlivening, seductive and sensual.

A unique, luxurious massage blend can be made by mixing neroli with rose, jasmine and ylang-ylang. Neroli is believed to regenerate skin cells, heal broken veins and improve skin elasticity. As a result, it is a popular ingredient in expensive skincare products.

Neroli can also be useful:

	Bereavement
	Hysteria
	Shock
	Fright
	Nerves about exams or a job interview
	Depression
	Tearfulness
	Disorientation
	Restlessness
	Stress
	Insomnia
	Anxiety
	Over-sensitivity
	Irritability

*"If you believe
in aromatherapy...
it works, if you
don't believe
in aromatherapy...
it works!"*

CRISTINA PROANO-CARRION

"You anoint my head with oils, my cup overflows."

PSALM 23:5

ORANGE

With the aroma of spring and summer, orange essential oil is warm and cheering. It is refreshing and brings lightness, happiness and positivity to all that use it. Its citrus fragrance smells like freshly grated orange peel. It is commonly used in cooking, adding a natural flavour to sweets, puddings and mulled wine.

Orange essential oil is perfect when you are guilty of taking things too seriously and forgetting to laugh!

Orange can also be useful for:

	Lack of energy
	Sadness
	Fear of the unknown
	Insomnia
	Irritability
	Self-consciousness
	Stubbornness
	Digestive complaints
	Depression
	Feelings of withdrawal
	Negativity
	Butterflies in the tummy
	Anxiety
	Boredom
	Selfishness

PALMAROSA

Palmarosa essential oil has a fresh, green, floral fragrance that has been likened to geranium and rose. It is often added to perfume, soaps and cosmetics as a substitute for rose.

Palmarosa is even sometimes used as a flavouring agent in tobacco! It blends well with bergamot, geranium, jasmine, patchouli, fennel, lavender, lime, melissa, orange, petitgrain, rose, ylang-ylang, rosewood, sandalwood and lemon.

Palmarosa can also be useful for:

	Loss of appetite
	Fevers
	Stomach pain
	Soothing the emotions
	Aching muscles and tendons
	Restlessness

PATCHOULI

With a musky, sweet fragrance that is quite persistent, patchouli is often used as a base for perfume. Its earthy, smoky and woody aroma gives it an exotic and mysterious aura. Patchouli is clarifying and grounding, which is useful if you are anxious or if you need to see things more clearly.

It is said to have aphrodisiac properties, and it can even function as an antidote to snake and insect bites.

Note: Patchouli should only be used in small doses, as too much can have a sedative effect.

Patchouli can also be useful for:

	Headaches
	Viruses
	Depression
	Apprehension
	Cracked skin
	Water retention
	Fevers
	Lethargy
	Anxiety
	Clarity
	Sores
	Cellulite

"Believe it or not, I am a big fan of patchouli oil. I know it's not a universally liked fragrance. I usually combine it with other essential oils – I have many mixtures I like."

OLIVIA WILDE

"*There is precious treasure and oil in the dwelling of the wise.*"

SOLOMON

PEPPERMINT

Cooling when warm and warming when cold, peppermint is refreshing, cleansing and stimulating. A must for any first-aid kit, it can help clear the head, stimulate the senses and fortify the body. Best known as a remedy for digestive upsets, peppermint is also ideal to use at the first hint of a cold. Peppermint can also be useful for:

	Aches and pains
	Ringworm
	Travel sickness
	Itchy skin
	Respiratory ailments
	Forgetfulness

	Hysteria
	Anger
	Loss of energy
	Shock
	Tired feet
	Nausea
	Scabies
	Headaches and migraines
	Neuralgia
	Digestive upsets
	Depression
	Mental fatigue
	Nervous trembling
	Loss of memory
	Faintness

PETITGRAIN

With an aroma that is fresh, light, floral and citrusy, petitgrain is often described as a slightly bitter version of neroli.

Petitgrain is a balancing type of oil that can relax and calm the subject while also uplifting the spirits.

Petitgrain can also be useful for:

	Calming a rapid heartbeat
	Easing breathing
	Skin blemishes and acne
	Soothing the emotions
	Insomnia
	Muscle spasms
	Digestive functions
	Depression
	Anger and panic attacks

PINE

Obtained from pine needles, this oil has a fresh, sharp, forest fragrance, so it is often used in cleaning products and disinfectants. It is necessary for every home during cold and flu season for purifying the environment and soothing respiratory ailments. Its strong curative properties were recognized by the ancient civilizations of Egypt, Greece and Arabia.

People with lung and breathing problems would flock to areas where pine trees grew to take advantage of the pure air. Native Americans used pine to repel fleas and lice and to prevent scurvy.

Pine can also be useful for:

	Bronchitis
	Digestive conditions
	Eczema
	Cuts and wounds
	Nervous exhaustion
	Hopelessness
	An overworked mind
	Respiratory complaints
	Painful, stiff joints and muscles
	Psoriasis
	Mental fatigue
	Depression
	Stress

ROSE

Considered the queen of the flowers, rose oil is the most expensive oil that can be bought in its pure form. As a result, most rose essential oils are diluted, often in grapeseed oil. The fragrance is quite intoxicating and manages to be both powerful and delicate. Rose oil is a renowned aphrodisiac which works on multiple levels. The sedative action of rose oil helps relieve nervous tension, balance emotions and uplift the mind, while also creating a sense of well-being. Rose can also be useful for:

	Allergies
	Addiction
	PMT and menstrual problems

	Fevers, coughs and sore throats
	Depression
	Attachment
	Fear
	Nerves
	Sadness
	Hangovers
	Migraines and headaches
	Circulation
	Gum disease
	Shingles
	Insomnia
	Bereavement and grief
	Regret
	Terror

ROSEMARY

This is an all-purpose oil; a well-deserved favourite of any aromatherapist. It helps restore mental clarity, gets rid of negativity and heals the body. Rosemary is penetrating and stimulating, with a strong, woody, herbal scent. It should be used sparingly, but blends well with basil, bergamot, cedarwood, grapefruit, lime and orange. *Note: If you are pregnant, have high blood pressure or epilepsy, you should avoid rosemary oil*. Otherwise, rosemary can be useful for:

	Chilblains
	Muscle ache and poor circulation
	Dandruff

	Migraines and hangovers
	High cholesterol
	Fainting and disorientation
	Oily skin
	Burns and wounds
	Cellulite
	Improving memory
	Poor digestion and constipation
	Tiredness
	Sneezing
	Arthritis
	Yeast infections
	Skin blemishes and acne
	Indecisiveness
	Sluggishness and lethargy

ROSEWOOD

Rosewood has a peppery, sweet and slightly floral aroma. It is so gentle that it is often used in skincare products. Rosewood oil is very versatile, and it blends well with many other oils.

The rosewood tree is an endangered species so you should consider the source of any rosewood oil that you buy.

Rosewood can be useful for:

	Coughs
	Bronchitis
	Acne

	Psoriasis
	Insect bites
	Convalescence
	Excessive daydreaming
	Instability
	Anxiety
	Tonsillitis
	Stress headaches
	Eczema
	Scarring
	Stings
	Apprehension and nervousness
	Grumpiness
	Depression
	Stress

SAGE

Sage essential oil promotes a calming and relaxing environment. It blends well with clary sage, bergamot, lemon and black pepper.

Note: Sage should be used in small quantities and is best administered by a qualified aromatherapist.

Sage can also be useful for:

	Improving memory
	Stress
	Depression
	Anxiety
	High cholesterol
	Can stimulate the metabolism
	Dandruff and oily hair

SANDALWOOD

Traditionally associated with self-expression, sandalwood has a woody, sweet aroma and is very versatile.

It is often used in incense, perfume and skincare. Sandalwood has emotional, spiritual and physical benefits, and it is also considered to be an aphrodisiac.

Sandalwood can also be useful for:

	Bronchitis
	Sinusitis
	Dry coughs
	Cystitis

	Catarrh
	Fear
	Depression
	Self-centredness
	Irritability
	Nerves
	Sore throats
	Tinnitus
	Loss of voice
	Eczema
	Cynicism
	Insecurity
	Stress
	Sensitivity
	Listlessness

TEA TREE

With a strong medicinal smell, tea tree essential oil is antibacterial, antifungal, and a stimulant for the immune system.

Tea tree oil is often described as "nature's first aid in a bottle". It helps the immune system to fight off disease, helps shorten the duration of illness and is useful in the cold and flu season.

Tea can also be used for:

	Thrush
	Herpes
	Glandular fever

	Toothache
	Warts
	Nappy rash
	Recovery after illness
	Nervous exhaustion
	Hysteria
	Mouth ulcers
	Verrucas
	Ringworm
	Spider and scorpion bites
	Athlete's foot
	Dry scalp and dandruff
	Chickenpox and shingles
	Spots and blemishes
	Shock

THYME

Thyme is a common herb that is used in cooking. As an essential oil, distilled from the flowers of the plant, thyme is a useful antibacterial.

Before a battle, Roman soldiers were said to bathe in thyme to make them more courageous. At the same time, the Egyptians used it for embalming dead bodies.

Note: Thyme oil is best administered by a professional aromatherapist.

Thyme can also be useful for:

	Improving blood circulation
	Strengthening the immune system
	Joint pain
	Cramps and spasms
	Acne
	Blood clots
	Digestive functions
	Throat infections
	Bacterial infections
	Chickenpox and measles scars

VETIVER

With an earthy, dense, musky smell, vetiver is often compared to myrrh and patchouli.

Its properties resemble that of the female hormone oestrogen, making it an appropriate choice during menopause, when the hormone needs supplementing.

Vetiver can also be useful for:

	Arthritis and rheumatism
	Moisturizing ageing skin
	Oversensitivity
	Emotional shock or trauma
	Nerves
	Aches and pains
	Skin
	Relaxation
	Anorexia
	Repelling moths

YLANG-YLANG

Ylang-ylang means "flower of flowers". Ylang-ylang has a sweet, soft, flowery and exotic aroma which conjures images of orchids and jasmine. This oil is a potent aphrodisiac that creates erotic and sensual moods. Conversely, ylang-ylang is also calming and relaxing, with sedative properties. This oil relaxes the body while elevating the spirits and can replace negativity with positivity. It can help several psychological conditions, including:

	Anger and jealousy
	Guilt
	Stubbornness
	Lack of self-esteem
	Irrationality
	Fear of people
	Stress and tension
	Impatience
	Detachment
	Panic attacks
	Suspiciousness
	Lack of self-confidence
	Shyness
	Nervous depression
	Insomnia

CHAPTER

3

TOP TIPS

"*Personally,
I don't use fragrance
and only use
essential oils.*"

DONNA KARAN

USEFUL
ESSENTIAL OILS

- **Lavender**
- **Tea tree**
- **Lemon**
- **Peppermint**
- **Eucalyptus**
- **Clove**
- **Chamomile**
- **Frankincense**
- **Grapefruit**
- **Oregano**

POPULAR ESSENTIAL OILS

- Lavender
- Bergamot
- Frankincense
- Peppermint
- Rosemary
- Geranium
- Ylang-ylang
- Tea tree
- Eucalyptus
- Clary sage

MOST EXPENSIVE ESSENTIAL OILS

Champaca absolute £1,840 ($2,380) per ounce

Tuberose absolute £1,341 ($1,733) per ounce

Frangipani absolute £1,208 ($1,561) per ounce

Cannabis flower £771 ($996) per ounce

Agarwood £693 ($895) per ounce

Rose £570 ($736)per ounce

Seaweed absolute £530 ($685) per ounce

Elecampane absolute £456 (589) per ounce

Sandalwood £400 ($517) per ounce

Neroli £288 ($372) per ounce

APHRODISIAC ESSENTIAL OILS

- Clary sage
- Lavender
- Sandalwood
- Ylang-ylang
- Black pepper
- Rose
- Jasmine
- Patchouli
- Ginger
- Cedarwood

STRESS-BUSTING ESSENTIAL OILS

- Lavender
- Bergamot
- Lemongrass
- Neroli
- Lemon
- Orange
- Ylang-ylang
- Frankincense
- Rose
- Chamomile

CHAPTER
4

BLENDING ESSENTIAL OILS

When two or more essential oils are blended together, they create a synergy, balancing each other and combining the therapeutic benefits of both. At first, use equal amounts of each, then you can experiment with different proportions as you become more experienced. You should always use a carrier oil, such as jojoba, grape or almond, if you are using your blend for massage or in the bath.
There are three ways in which you can blend essential oils:
by fragrance, by note or by effect.

*"We all have the ability
to heal ourselves; I know,
I have done so...
In the morning, know that
you are Loved, You Are Love
and You Love."*

LISA BELLINI

BLENDING by FRAGRANCE

You can combine any oils which have an aroma that you like; however, oils from the same group tend to blend really well. Essential oils can be divided roughly into five different fragrance groups, which are: citrus, floral, herbal, spicy and woody.

citrus

bergamot, grapefruit, lemon, neroli, orange

floral

rose, geranium, ylang-ylang

herbal

basil, chamomile, clary sage, eucalyptus,
marjoram, rosemary, tea tree, thyme

spicy

coriander, black pepper, cinnamon,
peppermint

woody

cedarwood, frankincense, cypress, juniper,
patchouli, sandalwood

BLENDING
by NOTE

Every essential oil has a "note", depending on how quickly they evaporate. Fragrances that fade the quickest are "top notes"; those that last the longest are "base notes"; and those in between are known as "middle notes". We usually smell top notes first, and they are generally floral or citrus oils. Base notes are more in-depth, heavier scents that are traditionally woody oils. In contrast, middle notes bind the two together and are typically herbs and spices.

A typical blend by note would consist of:
30% Top + 50% Middle + 20% Base oil

top notes
bergamot, grapefruit, lemon, lemongrass, orange, basil, eucalyptus

middle notes
lavender, rose, geranium, coriander, cinnamon, clove, cypress, chamomile, clary sage, marjoram, oregano, rosemary, tea tree, thyme

base notes
ylang-ylang, black pepper, cedarwood, frankincense, patchouli, sandalwood, peppermint

BLENDING by
EFFECT

Different oils and blends will have different effects on moods and on any physical conditions.

We can divide them into four groups which blend well together:

energizing

bergamot, grapefruit, lemon, lemongrass,
orange, coriander, black pepper, cinnamon,
clove, cypress, basil, clary sage, eucalyptus,
peppermint, rosemary, sage, tea tree

relaxing

bergamot, geranium, lavender,
ylang-ylang, cedarwood, frankincense,
patchouli, clary sage, sage,
thyme, rose

cleansing

grapefruit, lemon, orange, oregano,
patchouli, peppermint

grounding

bergamot, orange, rose, geranium, lavender,
coriander, black pepper, oregano, cedarwood,
frankincense, sandalwood, chamomile,
marjoram, thyme

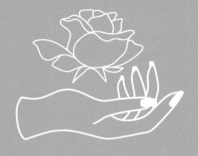

CHAPTER
5

UNUSUAL
SITUATIONS

In this chapter, we investigate the idea of using complementary therapies and aromatherapy in unusual situations. We also look at treating pets, along with horses.

You will find some suggestions for the use of aromatherapy around the house and for a holiday first-aid kit.

"With the increasing demand for holistic health care and the 'green revolution', the demand for aromatherapy will increase, and hopefully we will reach the point where medical doctors incorporate it into their repertoire."

ROBERT TISSERAND

AROMATHERAPY
during
PREGNANCY

I wouldn't advise anybody to use anything invasive while pregnant. The word "invasive" means something that *invades* the body, and we know that anything you put *onto* the skin will find its way *into* the body through the skin.

An excellent way of using aromatherapy while pregnant is by using a diffuser, either the little stick diffusers that release a small amount of essence into the air as the day goes by, or a pottery diffuser, where you put a tea-light candle inside and a drop of essential oil into a dish on top.

The candle warms the essence and allows the aroma to waft around the room.

Having said that, I would avoid using any kind of aromatherapy even in a diffuser if you have any of the following problems:

- A history of miscarriage
- Vaginal bleeding during the pregnancy
- Epilepsy
- Heart problems
- Diabetes
- Blood clotting problems
- Kidney or liver disease
- Are taking antibiotics or antihistamines

So, if you are in good health and you want to diffuse some essence, the following might be useful, in addition to being calming and relaxing.

Only ever use essential oils after three months of pregnancy have passed, and only use the following ones: neroli, tangerine, chamomile, lavender, peppermint and ylang-ylang.

AROMATHERAPY
during
CHILDBIRTH

Some hospitals have midwives who are specially trained in aromatherapy, and clinical trials have shown that the use of essential oils during childbirth may reduce the likelihood of the mother needing heavy-duty pain killers or an epidural.

If you decide to use aromatherapy, only do so with the aid of a fully qualified professional and only while in a hospital. Even so, I would not recommend putting any essential oil onto the body as a massage or in a bath. Anything put into a bath could travel through into the vagina and cause a reaction or an infection, or it could land on the emerging baby.

The following essential oils can be used in a diffuser during labour to boost contractions, reduce anxiety and ease pain: ginger, clary sage, mandarin, lavender, lemongrass, frankincense or chamomile.

BABIES
and INFANTS

I wouldn't recommend aromatherapy
for a baby or infant at all. Things that
are put *onto* the skin soon find their way
into the body, which, of course, is the
whole point of aromatherapy.

If your baby is unsettled, you must consult a medical professional, because he could have a hidden health problem.

If the baby has a clean bill of health but still has occasional periods of being unsettled (say, when teething), a cuddle and a bit of gentle stroking is the best treatment.

AROMATHERAPY
for
PETS

Important note: An animal can't tell you if it has an allergy or if it is reacting badly to something.

This reinforces my view that it is a bad idea to use anything directly on the skin of any animal.

Use a diffuser to waft a little of the essence around the area in which the animal spends some of its day, but make sure the diffuser is out of the animal's reach.

Dogs and horses respond well to aromatherapy treatment for physical, emotional and behavioural ailments. However, you must still check out the situation with your vet. You should also have exceptional knowledge of your pet's normal behaviour and character before using essential oils so that you can be alert to any unwanted side effects.

Important notes

- Cats have an exceptional sense of smell and a sensitive metabolic system, so an essential oil that might seem mild to us may be too intense and overwhelming for a cat, so it's best to avoid aromatherapy in any form for cats.

- Pet rodents and small mammals (gerbils, hamsters, rabbits, rats etc.) are too small to cope with what would be overwhelmingly strong medicine to them.

- Birds have a highly sensitive metabolic system, so birds and essential oils do not mix.

- Do not use aromatherapy in any form for fish and reptiles due to their pH levels and aquatic environments.

- If a pet is unwell, it is advised to take them to the vet but also give them lots of love.

useful
ESSENTIAL OILS
for DOGS

These are some aromatherapy oils
particularly suited to dogs:

cedarwood

Good for skin and dermatitis as cedarwood
is antiseptic and soothing. It also has flea-
repellent properties.

chamomile

Anti-inflammatory and gentle, chamomile is
ideal for soothing and calming nervous dogs. It
is also suitable for helping joint pain.

clary sage

A calming essence.

eucalyptus

An excellent essence for kennel cough or other
respiratory complaints, eucalyptus is antiviral
and anti-inflammatory.

geranium

Excellent for skin irritations and ear infections. Geranium is also an good tick repellent.

ginger

Perfect for anything sickness-related, such as travel sickness or an upset stomach.

lavender

A fantastic all-rounder that is excellent for skin irritation, anxiety, insect bites and travel sickness and for calming down a nervous or anxious dog.

marjoram

Insect-repellent, antibacterial, calming and relaxing.

peppermint

An excellent oil to soothe pain or sickness.

neroli

Can calm a dog as well as stimulate
their appetite.

thyme

Great for relieving pain such as arthritis
or rheumatism.

Important notes

- If your dog is ill, in pain, itchy or uncomfortable, you must take it to the vet and use whatever product they recommend.

- If your dog has fleas or ticks, buy a good-quality product with which to treat the dog. Also, consider using essential oils for cleaning and fragrancing your home to help repel fleas. Citronella, cedar, rosemary, peppermint, lemongrass and lavender can all help to prevent a flea infestation in the house.

Aromatherapy might be useful in the following cases:

- To calm down
- To reduce aggression
- To reduce hyperactivity
- To reduce barking
- To treat insect bites and stings
- To get rid of that "doggy" smell
- To treat bad breath
- To prevent travel sickness
- To reduce arthritic pain
- To treat dry skin
- To help with nervousness

AROMATHERAPY
for
HORSES

Aromatherapy can treat a host of ailments in horses – from sweet itch, muscular aches and mud fever through to nervousness and skittishness.

You must use a qualified equine aromatherapist who has been approved by your vet to administer any aromatherapy treatments to a horse.

Even a diffuser might be the wrong thing to use, so always consult your vet before doing anything.

AROMATHERAPY
around the
HOUSE

Essential oils do not need to be restricted to individuals.

They can be just as useful around the house, for cleaning purposes, while also smelling great.

BATHROOMS

Tea tree, oregano and eucalyptus oils are particularly effective when cleaning the bathroom.

They can be used in toilets, sinks and drains to help dispel viruses.

Pine is also an excellent germ killer for toilets.

BEDROOMS

Make a mattress spray with a blend of two or three of the oils listed below. Put a few drops in a bottle with some water and spray as needed. Not only will the bed smell nice but it will be free of germs, dust and bed mites. Lavender will also help you to get a good night's sleep.

- **Eucalyptus**
- **Lavender**
- **Tea tree**
- **Rosemary**

KITCHENS

Black pepper, bergamot, lemon, grapefruit and orange are all great ingredients for a multi-purpose kitchen cleaner. Again, add a few drops to a bottle of water and spray the mixture on kitchen surfaces.

Although not an essence as such, white vinegar is a truly excellent natural product that can be used for cleaning.

FLOORS

Lemon essential oil can dissolve dirt and marks from tiles and hardwood.

For a beautiful carpet deodorizer, combine sixteen ounces of baking powder with *one* of the following combinations:

- 30 drops of lavender oil

- 10 drops each of lime, lemon and orange essential oil

- 15 drops of spearmint oil and 10 drops of peppermint

- 15 drops of geranium and 5 drops of rosemary oil

- 10 drops each of chamomile, tea tree and rosemary essential oil

Put the blend into a container (a salt shaker is ideal) and apply liberally to carpets. Leave overnight or for at least two hours and then vacuum.

top tips for a holiday

FIRST-AID KIT

Take a carrier oil with you such as coconut, olive, jojoba or sweet almond. Although not an essential oil, a natural remedy for minor skin irritations is witch hazel, so it is worth taking some of this with you too.

Infections
Thyme, lavender, chamomile, eucalyptus, tea tree, oregano

Bites
Lavender, chamomile, eucalyptus, thyme

Insect repellent
Citronella, lemongrass, lavender, thyme, peppermint

Jetlag
Lemongrass, grapefruit, peppermint, lavender, eucalyptus, geranium

Heatstroke
    Lavender, eucalyptus, peppermint, chamomile
Travel sickness
    Ginger, peppermint
Toothache
    Peppermint, clove oil, chamomile
Wounds
    Lavender, chamomile, tea tree
Vomiting
    Peppermint, ginger, lavender, lemon juice
    in spring water with sweetener
Bruises
    Chamomile, geranium, lavender
Fevers
    Eucalyptus, peppermint, lavender
Insect bites
    Thyme, eucalyptus, chamomile, lavender
Constipation
    Peppermint, thyme
Colds
    Ginger, thyme, eucalyptus

CHAPTER

6

BLEND for DIFFERENT CONDITIONS

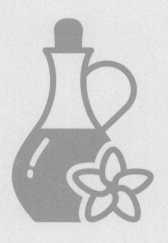

The following list shows the essences to use in a variety of conditions.

a

Acne: chamomile, tea tree, frankincense, lavender
Addiction: clary sage, rose
Allergies: rose, juniper
Anger: ylang-ylang, grapefruit, bergamot
Antibacterial: tea tree, rosemary
Anxiety: bergamot, rosemary
Apathy: jasmine, rosemary
Aphrodisiac: jasmine, ylang-ylang
Apprehension: frankincense, patchouli
Arthritis/rheumatism: chamomile, lavender,
    juniper, ginger
Asthma: cedarwood, cypress, eucalyptus

b

Bedwetting: chamomile, lavender, cypress
Bites: lavender, tea tree
Bitterness: grapefruit, lavender, ylang-ylang
Boredom: lemongrass, grapefruit, rosemary
Broken veins: neroli, lavender
Bronchitis: cedarwood, cypress, eucalyptus,
    sandalwood

Bruises: lavender, tea tree
Burns: tea tree, lavender

C

Chilblains: rosemary, sandalwood, chamomile, lavender
Clarity: grapefruit, rosemary
Claustrophobia: clary sage, frankincense
Circulation: rosemary, lavender
Colds: cinnamon, eucalyptus, ginger, cypress
Compulsiveness: clary sage, patchouli
Concentration: basil, lemongrass
Confidence: jasmine, ginger, bergamot, ylang-ylang
Confusion: cardamom, grapefruit
Constipation: rosemary, black pepper
Coughs: cypress, sandalwood
Courage: frankincense, jasmine
Cracked skin: frankincense, patchouli
Cramp: juniper, rosemary, marjoram, lemongrass
Cuts: lavender, tea tree

Cynicism: sandalwood, jasmine
Cystitis: juniper, sandalwood, lavender, eucalyptus

d

Dandruff: cypress, cedarwood, rosemary
Depression: bergamot, clary sage
Dermatitis: rosemary, chamomile, geranium,
    lavender
Despondency: bergamot, grapefruit
Detachment: jasmine, ylang-ylang
Disorientation: rosemary, neroli
Dry skin: geranium, sandalwood

e

Eczema: lavender, frankincense, geranium,
    chamomile
Exhaustion: clary sage, lavender, orange, basil,
    rosemary
Envy: grapefruit, rose

f

Fainting: basil, rosemary

Fear: frankincense, lavender, rose, jasmine, sandalwood, ylang-ylang
Flatulence: fennel, rosemary
Frustration: grapefruit, jasmine

g

Grief: rose, neroli, frankincense
Guilt: ylang-ylang, basil, sandalwood

h

Hangovers: rose, juniper, rosemary
Hayfever: juniper rose
Headache: lavender, peppermint, eucalyptus, basil, rosemary
Hostility: clary sage, marjoram, ylang-ylang
Hot flushes: chamomile, geranium
Hysteria: neroli, lavender

i

Indecisiveness: grapefruit, rosemary
Impatience: lavender, ylang-ylang
Insect bites/repellent: lavender, lemongrass

Insecurity: frankincense, lavender, sandalwood
Insomnia: clary sage, lavender
Irrationality: lavender, ylang-ylang, marjoram
Irritability: grapefruit, ylang-ylang, neroli, rose,
    frankincense, sandalwood, chamomile, lavender

m

Menopause: geranium, clary sage
Migraines: rose, juniper, lavender
Monday morning feeling: rosemary, bergamot
Mood swings: geranium, lavender
Muscle aches: lemongrass, rosemary, black
    pepper, cypress

n

Nausea: lavender, peppermint, fennel
Negative thoughts: bergamot, clary sage,
    lavender
Nerves: camphor, sandalwood, grapefruit,
    frankincense, rose
Nightmares: frankincense, clary sage, sandalwood
Nosebleeds: cypress, frankincense, lavender

o

Obsession: bergamot, clary sage, lavender
Over-thinking: clary sage, jasmine
Overwork: clary sage, marjoram, neroli, lavender,
   lemongrass, frankincense

p

Panic attacks: frankincense, lavender
Paranoia: lavender, frankincense
PMT: juniper, geranium, bergamot, lavender,
   rose
Psoriasis: bergamot, geranium, lavender
Procrastination: grapefruit, sandalwood

r

Regret: bergamot, rose
Rejuvenation: frankincense, rose
Relaxation: clary sage, lavender, marjoram
Respiratory tract infections: eucalyptus,
   pine, tea tree
Restlessness: chamomile, lavender, clary sage,
   neroli

Rigidity: geranium, jasmine ylang-ylang

S
Sadness: jasmine, rose
Self-criticism: frankincense, sandalwood, ylang-ylang
Self-esteem: sandalwood, ylang-ylang
Selfishness: lemon, orange, ylang-ylang
Sensitivity: juniper, sandalwood, ylang-ylang
Shivering: marjoram, rosemary
Shock: neroli, lavender
Shyness: bergamot, jasmine, ylang-ylang
Sluggishness: lemon, cypress, rosemary
Sickness: cinnamon, peppermint, black pepper, lavender, juniper, rose
Sinusitis: eucalyptus, lavender, basil, sandalwood
Sprains: lavender, chamomile
Stage fright: lavender, ylang-ylang
Stings: lavender, chamomile
Stress: cedarwood, clary sage, neroli
Stomachache: peppermint, chamomile

Sunburn: lavender, chamomile

t

Tantrums: chamomile, lavender
Teething: lavender, chamomile
Tendon pain: rosemary, lavender, juniper
Throat soreness: lavender, sandalwood
Throat infection: tea tree, thyme
Thrush: tea tree, thyme
Tinnitus: lavender, peppermint, sandalwood
Toothache: clove, peppermint
Too talkative: cypress, marjoram
Travel sickness: peppermint, lavender,
    bergamot, chamomile

V

Varicose veins: cypress, lavender

W

Worry: chamomile, lavender